The Plant Based C

Healthy, Easy and Quick Recipes for a Green, Whole-Food Diet

Penny Tripp

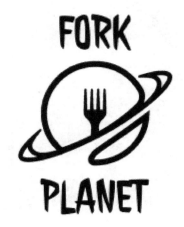

FORK

PLANET

Also by Penny Tripp

Penny Tripp Plant Based Cookbooks
Plant Based Cookbook: Healthy and Delicious Recipes for Everyday
Plant Based Cookbook for Beginners: Healthy Recipes to Lose Weight and Live Longer
The Plant Based Cookbook: Tasty and Healthy Recipes to Lose Weight and Live Better
The Plant Based Cookbook for Beginners: Healthy, Easy and Quick Recipes for a Green, Whole-Food Diet

Table of Contents

Introduction...1

1. Lemon Chickpea Orzo Soup 3

2. Cinnamon Applesauce Bread...5

3. Healthy Baked Beans 7

4. Chocolate chia pudding...9

5. Black Bean + Quinoa Burritos 11

6. Grilled Peach, Corn & Zucchini Quinoa Salad + Lemon-Basil Vinaigrette... 15

7. Baked Apple Oatmeal.. 19

8. Triple Berry Chia Seed Jam 21

9. Tempeh Chow Mein 23

10. Crispy Blackened Tofu with Kale + Quinoa 25

11. Super Seed Chocolate Oatmeal 29

12. Country Hash Browns with Sausage Gravy 31

13. Mint Chocolate Smoothie 33

14. Muesli 35

15. Pumpkin Spice Chia Pudding 37

16. Carrot Pancakes... 39

17. Kid-Friendly Panini 41

18. Ginger Pear Green Smoothie 43

19. Creamy Coconut Milk Oatmeal 45

20. Coconut Chia Pudding with Honey & Lime 47

21. Quinoa Breakfast Porridge with Sautéed Apples 49

22. Vegetarian Sushi Cups... 51

23. Butternut Mac And 'Cheese' With Smoky Shiitake 'Bacon.' 53

24. Rainbow Collard Wraps with Peanut Butter Dipping Sauce ... 55

25. Curried Quinoa Chickpea Burgers 57

26. Baked Apples.. 59

27. Blistered Shishito Peppers 61

28. Red Sangria.. 63

29. Almond Flour Crackers 65

30. Quick N' Healthy Veggie Pasta Salad 67

31. Vegan Queso... 69

32. Greek Quinoa Salad 71

33. Pozole (Posole Verde) 73

34. Farro (No-Fuss Recipe) 75

35. American Goulash 77

36. Roasted Butternut Squash Salad 79

37. Cornbread 81

38. Macaroni Salad 83

39. Cream Cheese 85

40. Radish and Cucumber Salad 87

41. Apple, Beet, Carrot & Kale Salad 89

42. Portobello Fajitas 91

43. Baked Sweet Potato Wedges 93

44. Sonoma Chickpea 'Chicken' Salad 95

45. Balela Salad 97

46. Banana Boats 99

47. Spanish Vegan Paella 101

48. Kale + Red Cabbage Slaw 103

49. Hummus Veggie Wrap 105

50. Raw Ginger Snaps 107

Conclusion 109

Introduction

What is a Plant-Based Diet?

Plant-based is a wide phrase that refers to any diet that emphasizes non-animal plant-based foods such as whole grains, legumes, nuts, fruits, and vegetables. Vegan and vegetarian diets and individuals who aim to consume meat only once or twice a week are examples of this. Whether you are vegan or just trying to eat less meat, almost 87 percent of Americans don't receive their daily vegetable portions, so focusing on eating more vegetables is a smart idea.

A whole-food, plant-based diet is based on the following concepts and allows you to fulfill your nutritional requirements by concentrating on natural, minimally processed plant foods:

Natural, less processed foods are referred to as "whole foods." This refers to substances that are entire, unprocessed, or little processed.

Plant-based food is defined as food made entirely of plants and does not include animal products, including meat, eggs, milk, or honey.

A precise definition of what constitutes a whole-foods, plant-based diet is lacking (WFPB diet). The WFPB diet is more of a way of life than a strict dietary regimen.

This is because plant-based diets may vary significantly depending on how many animal items are included in a person's diet.

Nonetheless, the following are the fundamental concepts of a whole-foods, plant-based diet:

Whole, less processed meals are emphasized. Animal products are limited or avoided. Plants, such as vegetables, fruits, legumes, whole grains, seeds, and nuts, should account for the bulk of your diet. Refined foods, such as added sugars, white flour, and processed oils, are excluded.

A plant-based diet may be beneficial to your health as well as your intellect.

While the researchers found that this diet helps increase metabolism, weight management, and decrease inflammation (particularly in individuals with obesity and type 1 and type 2 diabetes), they could not confirm whether it improves mental performance.

Switching to a plant-based diet is one of the most effective ways to enhance your health, increase energy, and avoid chronic illnesses.

This cookbook series includes some amazing recipes, prepared using some of the best whole, hearty and healthy ingredients. All recipes are created by adding a few extra touches.

The dishes presented in this book are aimed at all members of the family and include everything from breakfast to lunch, snacks to dessert, and mouthwatering dinners. Enjoy!

1. Lemon Chickpea Orzo Soup

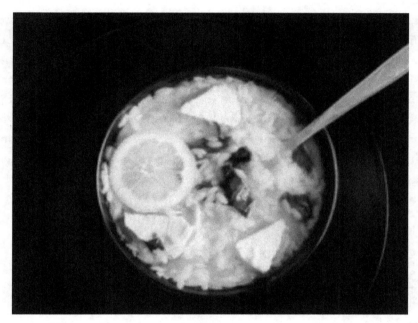

Preparation Time: 10 mins
Serves: 4

Ingredients:

- Chopped fresh dill, to taste
- Olive oil 1 tablespoon
- Onion, diced 1/2
- Carrots, 3 peeled and diced
- Garlic, minced 3 cloves
- Vegetable broth 7 – 8 cups
- Whole wheat orzo 1 cup

- Chickpeas (garbanzo beans), 2 cans (15oz.) Drained and rinsed
- Tahini 1/3 cup
- Lemon juice 1/4 – 1/2 cup (about 2 – 4 large lemons)
- Fresh baby kale or spinach a large handful

Method:
Over medium heat, heat the oil or water, add the onion and carrot, sauté for 5–7 minutes, add the garlic, and cook for 1 minute longer. Bring the broth or water to a boil, add the orzo or chickpeas, decrease the heat to medium-low, and simmer for 8 to 9 minutes, or until the orzo is cooked. Remove from the fire and whisk in the tahini & lemon juice (start with a tiny quantity of juice and add more to taste). Add the baby kale or spinach and toss well; the greens will soften & wilt in a matter of minutes. Season with salt and pepper and as much dill as you prefer. When the soup has sat for a while, it will thicken, so add extra liquids as required. Serve in separate bowls with crusty artisan bread to mop up all of the delicious juices. Enjoy!

Nutrition:
Calories: 196 kcal
Fats: 3.9 g
Proteins: 6.5 g
Carbs: 34.8 g

2. Cinnamon Applesauce Bread

Preparation Time: 5 mins
Serves: 10

Ingredients:

- Vanilla, optional 1 teaspoon
- Light spelt flour 2 cups
- Old fashioned oats, 1/2 cup optional
- Baking powder 2 teaspoons
- Baking soda 1/2 teaspoon
- Cinnamon 2 teaspoons
- Allspice 1/2 teaspoon
- Nutmeg 1/4 teaspoon
- Unsweetened applesauce 1 1/2 cups
- Maple syrup 1/2 cup
- Unsweetened almond milk 1/4 cup

Method:
Preheat the oven to 350 °F. Lightly grease or line a 9 x 5 loaf pan along with parchment paper.
Toss together the dry ingredients: Combine the flour, baking soda, oats, baking powder, cinnamon, nutmeg, allspice, and salt in a medium/large mixing basin.
Mix with the wet ingredients: Toss the dry ingredients with applesauce, maple syrup, & milk until barely incorporated. Take care not to overmix.
Bake: Pour mixture into prepared loaf pan, sprinkle with a handful of whole or quick oats if desired, and bake in the oven for 55 minutes. Allow cooling

completely before slicing. Enjoy!

Nutrition:
Calories: 211 kcal
Fats: 0.5 g
Proteins: 5 g
Carbs: 47.5 g

3. Healthy Baked Beans

Preparation Time: 10 mins
Serves: 6-8

Ingredients:

- Bay leaves 2
- Water 1/4 cup
- Onion, diced 1 medium
- Smoked paprika 2 teaspoons
- Garlic powder 1 heaping teaspoon
- Dried white beans 1 1b.
- SmallVegetable broth 4 cups low-sodium
- Pure maple syrup 1/3 cup
- Tomato paste 1/4 cup
- Apple cider vinegar 1/4 cup
- Mustard 2 tablespoons
- Fresh ground pepper 1/2 teaspoon

Optional add-ins:

- Unsulfured blackstrap molasses 2 – 4 tablespoons
- Jalapeno
- Green bell pepper

Method:
Add 1/4 cup water to the SAUTE setting on your Instant Pot. When the pan is
heated, add the onion and cook for 4 minutes. Cook, constantly stirring, for 1

minute, or till aromatic, after adding the smoked paprika & garlic powder. After that, carefully whisk in the beans, broth, apple cider vinegar, tomato paste, maple syrup, mustard, bay leaves, pepper until the tomato paste is completely dissolved and everything is properly incorporated. Place the lid on top, & make sure the vent is set to seal. Manually set the PRESSURE COOKER to HIGH for 75 minutes after pressing the PRESSURE COOKER button. Allow 20 minutes for the steam to escape. Move the vent to the open position, being cautious not to burn yourself if there is still any steam present. Remove the cover and let it cool slightly before seasoning with salt to taste. Transfer the beans to a serving dish after removing the bay leaves. Once the beans have cooled, they will thicken. If the mixture is too thick, add water at a time, stirring well after each addition, until the appropriate consistency is achieved. Enjoy!

Nutrition:
Calories: 119 kcal
Fats: 0.5 g
Proteins: 6 g
Carbs: 27 g

4. Chocolate chia pudding

Preparation Time: 4 hr.
Serves: 4

Ingredients:

- Vanilla extract 2 teaspoons
- Unsweetened almond milk 2 cups
- Chia seeds 1/4 cup + 2 tablespoons 100% cocoa/cacao powder 1/3 cup
- Pure maple syrup 1/4 – 1/3 cup

Method:
Whisk together the milk, chia seeds, maple syrup, cocoa powder, vanilla, and salt in a medium mixing bowl until well combined. Be patient; blending in the cocoa powder will take about a minute. Cover and chill in the refrigerator. After 30 minutes, give it a thorough stir (this step is critical. Otherwise, your pudding will not set correctly, and you'll end up with a soupy mixture), cover, and chill again. After 15 to 30 minutes, give it another stir. Within 4 hours, the pudding must be thickened & ready to serve, and after 8–10 hours, it will be at its thickest. Enjoy!

Nutrition:
Calories: 113.7 kcal
Fats: 10 g
Proteins: 5.4 g
Carbs: 12.5 g

5. Black Bean + Quinoa Burritos

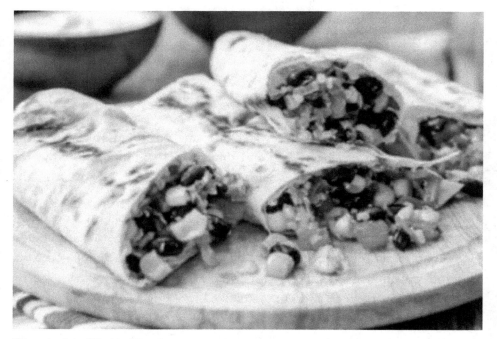

Preparation Time: 15 mins
Serves: 6-8

Ingredients:

- Tortillas 6 – 8 medium/large
- Dried quinoa 1/2 cup
- Water 3/4 cup + 1
- Olive oil 1 tablespoon
- Red onion, diced 1/2 large
- Orange bell pepper, 1 seeds removed and diced

- Diced tomatoes, 1 can (14oz) drained
- Zucchini, diced 1 medium
- Black beans, 2 cans (14 oz) drained and rinsed
- Corn, drained 1 can (14 oz)
- Cilantro, roughly chopped 1/4 – 1/2 cup
- Cumin 2 teaspoons
- Chili powder 1 teaspoon
- Chipotle powder 3/4 – 1 teaspoon
- Garlic powder 1 teaspoon
- Onion powder 1/2 teaspoon

Method:

Quinoa: Combine the quinoa & water in a small/medium saucepan, bring to a boil, cover, lower heat to low, and simmer for 13 minutes. Remove the cover and set aside for 10 minutes before fluffing with a fork. Remove from the equation.

Filling: Heat oil/water in a big skillet or pot on medium heat, add onion & sauté for 4 minutes, add bell pepper and simmer for another 2 minutes. Cook for another 3 mins or so after adding the tomatoes, zucchini, and corn. Continue to simmer until the black beans, chipotle, garlic, quinoa, cilantro, cumin, & onion powder, and salt are cooked through. Put tortillas on a flat surface, top with a mound of filling, allowing space all the way around, fold it in half, fold up every end, & roll the burrito away from you to seal it fully. Saran wrap, Freeze using foil, freezer paper or whatever you're accustomed to using for freezing. To minimize freezer burn, consume the paper sandwich bags within a few weeks if using them. They aren't likely to last that long! Warm in the toaster oven at 375 °F for 10 minutes or in the microwave for 30 seconds if at room temperature. If frozen, reheat in a 375°F oven for 30 minutes or in the microwave for 1:30–2 minutes. Serve it with sliced avocado & salsa of your choice. Enjoy!

Nutrition:
Calories: 657.7 kcal

Fats: 17.4 g
Proteins: 34.1 g
Carbs: 95.1 g

6. Grilled Peach, Corn & Zucchini Quinoa Salad + Lemon-Basil Vinaigrette

Preparation Time: 15 mins
Serves: 6

Ingredients:

- Pepitas (pumpkin seeds) small handful
- Dried quinoa 1 cup
- Water 1 3/4 cups
- Peaches 2 (ripe but firm)
- Corn on the cob 2
- Zucchini 2 medium
- Cherry tomatoes 1 cup
- Chickpeas 1 can (15 oz)
- Avocado 1/2

Lemon-Basil Vinaigrette:

- Red pepper flakes pinch
- Packed basil leaves 1/4 – 1/3 cup
- Olive oil 3 – 4 tablespoons
- Lemon juice 2 tablespoons (about 1 medium lemon)
- Apple cider vinegar 2 – 3 teaspoons
- Garlic, chopped 1 small clove

Method:

Quinoa: Combine quinoa, water, and vegetable broth in a medium pot. Bring to a simmer, then lower to low heat and cook for 15 minutes. Remove the cover and set it aside for 10 minutes before fluffing with a fork.

Vinaigrette: In a small/personal food processor, combine all ingredients and process until smooth and creamy. Alternately, finely chop the basil & mince the garlic, then whisk together all of the ingredients in a separate container – or toss the basil into the salad and whisk together the other vinaigrette ingredients. Set aside for a few minutes to allow the flavors to meld. To modify the flavor, taste again before combining. If you're preparing it a day or two ahead of time, keep it refrigerated. Remove any husks from the corn, take them away, knot them, and remove any silk threads from below. Cut peaches around the seam and twist the halves of the pit. Zoodles should be cut in half lengthwise. If desired, brush the cut sides of the peaches or zucchini with a small coating of oil before setting them on the grill; however, I did not do so since I greased the grill directly. Prepare your grill by brushing it with a thin layer of oil. Start with the corn since it will take the longest, around 10 minutes, depending on your grill. Then, cut side down, add the zucchini and peaches. The remaining two should cook in around 3–5 minutes on the grill. My pasta is al dente. Remove off the corn from the cob by shucking and slicing it. Holding the corn by its top horizontally in the middle of a large, shallow, rimmed baking dish like a pie dish, use a knife to gently but firmly chop the corn off the cob from top to bottom. Turn the corn 90 degrees and continue until all of the corn has been extracted. Using a vegetable slicer, cut zucchini into 1/4 - 1/2 inch slices. Peaches should be cut into 1/8 - 1/4 inch pieces. Half-cut the tomatoes. Half an avocado, twist to split halves, remove the seed, and thinly slice. Toss the quinoa with peaches, corn, chickpeas, zucchini, tomatoes, avocado, and pepitas in a large mixing bowl to incorporate. Mix in the dressing one more. To taste, season with mineral salt and freshly cracked pepper. Serve refrigerated or at room temperature. Serve plain or with a bunch of arugula on top. Enjoy!

Nutrition:
Calories: 458 kcal
Fats: 17.1 g

Proteins: 15.8 g
Carbs: 66.7

7. Baked Apple Oatmeal

Preparation Time: 5 mins
Serves: 6

Ingredients:

- Walnuts, chopped 1/2 – 1 cup
- Old-fashioned oats 2 cups
- Cinnamon 2 teaspoons
- Nutmeg 1/2 teaspoon
- Baking powder 1 teaspoon
- Unsweetened almond milk 2 cups
- Mashed banana, 1 cup optional
- Pure maple syrup, 1/4 cup optional
- Vanilla extract 1 teaspoon
- Apple 1 medium

Method:
Preheat the oven to 350 degrees Fahrenheit. If desired, lightly coat your baking dish with coconut oil. Mix the oats, cinnamon, baking powder, nutmeg, and salt in an 8-inch baking dish. Whisk together the milk, banana, optional syrup, and vanilla extract. Add chopped apples & walnuts to the top, mixing them in if desired. Preheat the oven to 350°F and bake for 30 mins on the center rack. Allow cooling slightly after completion. Slice and serve heated in individual bowls with desired toppings. Enjoy this tasty and well-worth-the-wait oatmeal. Enjoy!

Nutrition:
Calories: 374.3 kcal
Fats: 15.5 g
Proteins: 7.6 g
Carbs: 55.8 g

8. Triple Berry Chia Seed Jam

Preparation Time: 5 mins
Serves: 1

Ingredients:

- Pure maple syrup, 1 tablespoon optional
- Blackberries 1 heaping cup
- Raspberries 1/2 heaping cup
- Blueberries 1/2 heaping cup
- Chia seeds 1 heaping tablespoon

Method:
Combine the berries in a small skillet on the stovetop and cook over medium heat, turning periodically until softened. Mash the berries down the edge (or bottom) of the pan using the back of a slotted spoon or fork. Bring the mixture to a low boil. The cooking time would be between 4 and 6 minutes. Remove from fire after it reaches a boil, add sweetness if desired, and whisk in the chia seeds gently. Fill the jar with the mixture and set it aside to cool for a few minutes. To thicken, cover and store in the refrigerator. Refrigerate any leftovers. It will last 2–3 weeks. In a blender/food processor, combine the berries and chia seeds and pulse till desired chunkiness/consistency is achieved. Blend in as much maple syrup as required. Fill the jar with the mixture, cover it, and store it in the refrigerator to chill for a few hours. Keep your raw chia jam in the fridge & then use it within a week. Enjoy!

Nutrition:
Calories: 38 kcal
Fats: 0.1 g
Proteins: 0.8 g
Carbs: 2.4 g

9. Tempeh Chow Mein

Preparation Time: 10 mins
Serves: 4

Ingredients:

- White onion, sliced 1 small
- Chow mein noodles 8 – 12 oz.
- Package Tempeh 2 (8oz.)
- Packages Sesame oil 1 tablespoon
- Green cabbage 1/2 head (about 4 cups), shredded
- Celery stalk, 1 large sliced diagonally
- Carrots 2

Sauce:

- Ginger, minced 1 inch knob
- Tamari, coconut aminos 1/4 cup
- Pure maple syrup 2 tablespoons
- Water 2 tablespoons
- Rice wine vinegar, 1 tablespoon optional
- Garlic, minced 2 cloves

Method:
Noodles: Bring a pot of water to a boil, add chuka soba or chow mein noodles, reduce heat to medium, and cook for 4 minutes. Set aside after draining and rinsing. If you're using other noodles, follow the package directions for cooking. Stir together the ingredients for stir-fry sauce in a small bowl and set aside.

Tempeh + onion: Heat olive oil in a large wok over medium-high heat, crumble tempeh between your fingers, as well as cook for 2 minutes. Add the celery, cabbage, and carrot to the remaining vegetables and pour the sauce over them. Stir-fry for another 5–7 minutes, till the cabbage, has shrunk down as well as softened, stirring occasionally. Add the noodles and the remaining sauce to the vegetables, stir to coat, and heat until the noodles are warmed through. Season it with more tamari or other seasonings to taste. Serve it warm in individual bowls with scallions, red pepper flakes, and cilantro, if desired. Enjoy!

Nutrition:
Calories: 489 kcal
Fats: 8.2 g
Proteins: 32.7 g
Carbs: 73.4 g

10. Crispy Blackened Tofu with Kale + Quinoa

Preparation Time: 15 mins
Serves: 4

Ingredients:

Quinoa:

- Garlic powder 1/2 teaspoon
- Dried quinoa 1 cup
- Water 1 3/4 cups

Blackened Tofu:

- Olive oil 1 tablespoon
- Organic tofu, 1 block (14-16 oz) super firm
- Tamari, coconut amino's 2 tablespoons

Spice Blend:

- Cayenne pepper 1/8 teaspoon
- Paprika 2 teaspoons
- Black pepper 1/2 teaspoon
- Cornstarch, optional 1 teaspoon
- Garlic powder 1 teaspoon
- Onion powder 1 teaspoon
- Thyme 1 teaspoon
- Oregano 1/2 teaspoon

Sauteed Kale:

- Olive oil 1 tablespoon
- Chopped kale
- Nutritional yeast 2 tablespoons
- Garlic powder 1/2 teaspoon

Method:

Quinoa: To eliminate dust, rinse your quinoa under cold running water. Bring quinoa, garlic powder, a touch of salt, and water to a boil in a medium saucepan. Reduce heat to low, cover, and cook for 15 minutes. Cover, whisk and put aside for 10 mins to cool and absorb any extra liquid. Before serving, fluff the rice. It'll be fluffy and sprouted quinoa perfection.

Tofu prep: Tofu should be opened and drained.4 huge slabs of tofu (or whatever size you like). To remove extra moisture, press tofu between paper towels or a kitchen cloth. Place the tofu with tamari in a shallow dish and leave aside while preparing the blackening seasoning; flip after a few mins to let the other side soak.

Blackened Seasoning: Combine allspice blend ingredients in a medium-sized flat-bottomed mixing basin and stir until well combined. Because this dish is somewhat hot, you may choose to use less black pepper or cayenne. Place tofu slices in the spice mixture, gently press to obtain a nice covering, then flip and repeat on another side.

Cook tofu: Heat the oil in a saute pan over medium-high heat, then add the coated tofu and cook for 5 minutes on each side.

Sauteed Kale: Heat the oil in a big wok or saute pan over medium heat, add the kale and cook for 2 minutes, tossing constantly. Sprinkle the nutritional yeast & garlic powder on top, tossing and pushing the kale around to distribute the spices evenly. Stir fry for another four to five minutes, or until the spinach is brilliant green and barely wilted. In between stir-frying, you may cover the pan for a minute or two to help soften the kale. When the kale gets brilliant green, it's time to take it off the fire. Test a piece to check whether it's to your taste; if not, continue to sauté. Some people want it crisp, while others prefer it softer. Enjoy!

Nutrition:
Calories: 294 kcal
Fats: 11.8 g
Proteins: 16.9 g
Carbs: 32.7 g

11. Super Seed Chocolate Oatmeal

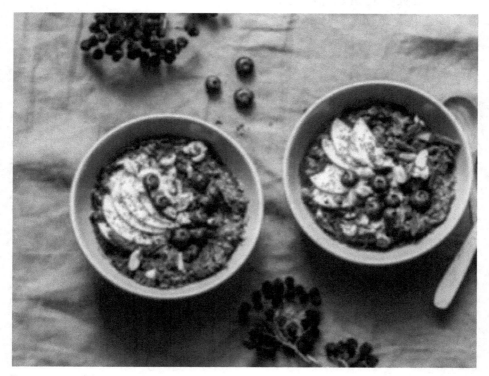

Preparation Time: 10 mins
Serves: 4 people

Ingredients:

- Date syrup (optional) 4 teaspoons
- Old fashioned oats 1 cup
- Water 2 cups
- Vanilla extract 1 teaspoons
- Ceylon cinnamon 1/2 tablespoon

- Cacao powder (or cocoa) 1 tablespoon
- Salt (optional) 1/4 teaspoon
- Ground flaxseeds 4 tablespoons
- Chia seeds 4 tablespoons
- Hemp seeds 2 tablespoons
- Walnuts 4 tablespoons
- Mixed organic berries 2 cups
- Plant yogurt 1/2 cup

Method:

In a saucepan, heat the water over medium-high heat. Heat until just boiling, then add the vanilla, chocolate, cinnamon, and salt. Once the water has heated up, the chocolate will mix in nicely. Stir in the oats until they are evenly distributed. Before boiling the water, add the oats for creamier oatmeal. Reduce to low heat and continue to whisk continuously for approximately 10 minutes. Defrost berries in a ceramic dish in the microwave for approximately 1 minute while the oats are heating.1/4 of the cooked oats should be added to each bowl. 1 tablespoon flax, 1 tablespoon chia seeds, and 1/2 tablespoon hemp seeds are sprinkled on top. These may also be added to the oats towards the end of the cooking process with approximately 1/4 cup of water. For each bowl, add 2 teaspoons of plant yogurt. If you like it sweeter, add berries, walnuts, and a teaspoon of date syrup. Enjoy!

Nutrition:
Calories: 354 kcal
Fats: 18.7 g
Proteins: 11.1 g
Carbs: 37.8 g

12. Country Hash Browns with Sausage Gravy

Preparation Time: 30 mins
Serves: 4

Ingredients:

Easy Gravy:

- Low sodium tamari 2 tsp
- Vegan breakfast sausage 1/3 lb. Cut into small pieces
- Whole wheat 3 tbsp
- Onion Powder 1/2 tsp
- Nutritional yeast 2 tbsp
- Vegetable broth 1 cup low-sodium
- Unsweetened milk 1 cup non-dairy

Hash Browns:

- Hash browns no added oil 1 lb. Frozen
- Onion diced 1/2
- Bell pepper 1
- Garlic minced 2 cloves
- Jalapeño (optional)
- 1 small Chives for garnish

Method:

In a medium non-stick pan, brown the vegan sausage over medium heat. Combine the flour, onion powder, salt, nutritional yeast, and pepper on top of the sausage. Whisk together the veggie broth, non-dairy milk, plus tamari or soy sauce. Continue to whisk over low heat till the gravy thickens. Reduce the heat and stay warm. Over medium heat, heat a large nonstick skillet. Spread the frozen hash browns evenly over the pan and cook for 6-10 minutes, then turn and cook for another 5 minutes, or until they begin to brown. Stir in the diced onion, garlic, and bell pepper until everything is well combined. Re-flatten the potatoes and veggies in an equal layer and set aside to brown again. Continue to turn and brown the hash browns till they are crispy to your liking. Serve the hash with a dollop of breakfast gravy and chives on top. Enjoy!

Nutrition:
Calories: 236 kcal
Fats: 4.8 g
Proteins: 11 g
Carbs: 39 g

13. Mint Chocolate Smoothie

Preparation Time: 5 mins
Serves: 2

Ingredients:

- Old fashioned oats 1/2 cup
- Bananas 4 medium cut into about 1" pieces and frozen
- Non-dairy milk 1/2 cup or more
- Fresh mint 1/2 cup lightly packed
- Spinach 2 handfuls
- Ground flaxseeds 1 tbsp
- Cacao nibs 2-3 tbsp

Method:
In the base of a high-powered blender, combine the optional oats, ground flax, and cacao nib. Combine the bananas, greens, and non-dairy milk in a blender. If you want additional cacao pieces, preserve them and add them after mixing the mixture a little more. Begin blending on low and gradually increase the speed. If the mixture is too thick, add additional non-dairy milk. Enjoy!

Nutrition:
Calories: 418 kcal
Fats: 12 g
Proteins: 8.3 g
Carbs: 74.8 g

14. Muesli

Preparation Time: 20 mins
Serves: 8

Ingredients:

- Almond extract 1 teaspoon
- Old fashioned oats 2 cups
- Wheat flakes uncle sam's brand 1 cup
- Quinoa flakes 1 cup
- Hemp hearts 1/2 cup
- Ground flaxseeds 1/2 cup
- Slivered almonds 1/2 cup
- Raw pumpkin seeds 1/2 cup
- Walnuts 1/2 cup
- Coconut flakes 1/2 cup
- Raisins 1/2 cup
- Ceylon cinnamon 1 teaspoon

Method:
In a large mixing basin, add all ingredients and whisk to blend. Keep in a tight-fitting glass jar or container. Serve with non-dairy milk, soy yogurt, and fruit. Enjoy!

Nutrition:
Calories: 430 kcal
Fats: 24 g

Proteins: 15.3 g
Carbs: 43 g

15. Pumpkin Spice Chia Pudding

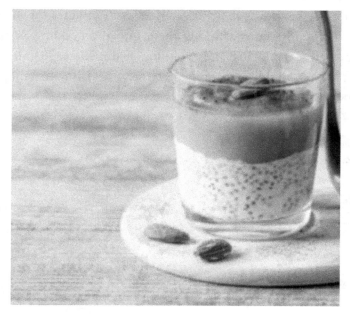

Preparation Time: 20 mins
Serves: 4

Ingredients:

- Pumpkin seeds 1 tbsp chopped walnuts or pecans
- Unsweetened almond milk 2 cups
- Pumpkin puree 1 cup
- Almond butter 2 tbsp
- Vanilla extract 1 tsp
- Maple syrup 1/4 cup
- Pumpkin pie spice 2 tsp

- Chia seeds 1/2 cup

Method:
In a glass dish, combine 1 cup almond milk and pumpkin puree. Stir in the puree until it is fully dissolved.Whisk together the almond butter, maple syrup, vanilla, and pumpkin spice until well combined.Whisk in the remaining almond milk before adding the chia seeds.Allow 5 minutes for the chia seeds to absorb the liquid before whisking them into the pudding.Refrigerate for 15 minutes before removing and whisking again.Allow 30 minutes in the refrigerator for the pudding to set.If preferred, garnish with pumpkin seeds, walnuts, coconut, or miniature chocolate chips. Enjoy!

Nutrition:
Calories: 205 kcal
Fats: 12 g
Proteins: 6.2 g
Carbs: 21.2 g

16. Carrot Pancakes

Preparation Time: 15 mins
Serves: 12 pancakes

Ingredients:

- Maple syrup or applesauce
- Old fashioned oats 1 cup
- Whole wheat flour 1/2 cup
- Cornmeal 1/4 cup
- Sea salt 1/2 tsp
- Ceylon cinnamon 1 tsp
- Baking soda 1 tsp
- Baking powder 1 tsp
- Ground flaxseeds 1 tbsp (optional)
- Carrot peeled and grated 1 large
- Banana mashed 1/2 large
- Vanilla extract 1 tsp
- Non-dairy milk 1 3/4 cup

Method:

In a large mixing bowl, combine all of the dry ingredients. Stir in the shredded carrots. In a mixing dish, combine the wet ingredients: almond, vanilla extract, and mashed banana. Stir everything together well. Allow for a 5-minute rest period. If the mixture is too thick, add additional liquid to thin it up. Preheat a nonstick skillet. If you're using a metal pan, a little coat of oil is required. When the pan is hot, put big spoonfuls of the pancake batter into it and cook until the bottoms are gently browned. Cook the opposite side as well. Serve with the remaining banana slices or blueberries, as well as maple syrup and applesauce. Enjoy!

Nutrition:
Calories: 119 kcal
Fats: 5.1 g
Proteins: 5 g
Carbs: 18.6 g

17. Kid-Friendly Panini

Preparation Time: 5 mins
Serves: 1

Ingredients:

- Whole grain bread 2 slices
- Raisins ¼ cup
- Hot water ¼ cup
- Cinnamon 1 tbsp
- Cacao powder 2 tsp
- Natural peanut butter ¼ cup
- Ripe banana 1

Method:
Combine the raisins, boiling water, cinnamon, and cacao powder in a mixing bowl. On whole-grain toast, spread peanut butter. Slice a banana and put it on top of a slice of peanut butter toast. Blend the raisin mixture and distribute it over the bread. Enjoy!

Nutrition:
Calories: 850 kcal
Fats: 34 g
Proteins: 27 g
Carbs: 112 g

18. Ginger Pear Green Smoothie

Preparation Time: 10 mins
Serves: 2

Ingredients:

- Vanilla extract 1/2 tsp
- Almond milk, unsweetened 2 cups
- Baby spinach 3 cups
- Ripe pears, 2 medium-sized cored
- Avocado chunks 1/2 cup (ideally frozen)
- Hemp seeds 2 tbsp
- Chia seeds 2 tbsp
- Ground ginger 1/2 tsp
- Ground cinnamon 1/2 tsp

Method:
Put all of the ingredients in a high-powered blender, starting with the almond milk. Blend for 1-2 minutes on high, or till smooth and creamy. If you like your smoothie to be a little runnier, add a little more almond milk. Enjoy right now or save for later. Enjoy!

Nutrition:
Calories: 377 kcal
Fats: 18 g
Proteins: 10 g
Carbs: 47 g

19. Creamy Coconut Milk Oatmeal

Preparation Time: 5 mins
Serves: 2

Ingredients:

- Maple syrup 1 tsp
- Rolled oats 1 cup
- Chia seeds 2 Tbsp
- Cinnamon 1/2 tsp
- Cardamom 1/4 tsp
- Canned coconut milk 1 cup
- Water 1 cup
- Vanilla extract 1 tsp

Method:

In a large pot on the stovetop, combine the oats, cinnamon, chia seeds, cardamom, and a sprinkle of salt. Combine the ingredients in a mixing bowl. Combine the coconut milk, vanilla extract, water, plus maple syrup in a mixing bowl. Bring the ingredients to a boil, then lower to low heat to keep them warm. Allow to simmer for approximately 5 mins, or till the liquid has been absorbed, stirring regularly. If you like thinner oats, alter the quantity of liquid. Toppings may be added to the oatmeal as desired. Enjoy while it's still hot. Enjoy!

Nutrition:
Calories: 284 kcal

Fats: 11 g
Proteins: 6 g
Carbs: 42 g

20. Coconut Chia Pudding with Honey & Lime

Preparation Time: 10 mins
Serves: 3

Ingredients:

- Chia seeds 6 Tbsp
- Honey 1 Tbsp
- 1/2 a lime, juice only
- Canned coconut milk 2 cups

Method:
Stir coconut milk, honey, chia seeds, and lime juice in a large mixing dish or jar until thoroughly blended. Refrigerate for 2 hours or overnight after covering the bowl/jar. Remove the chia pudding from the fridge and whisk it again. As desired, serve with additional toppings. Enjoy!

Nutrition:
Calories: 220 kcal
Fats: 13 g
Proteins: 4 g
Carbs: 20 g

21. Quinoa Breakfast Porridge with Sautéed Apples

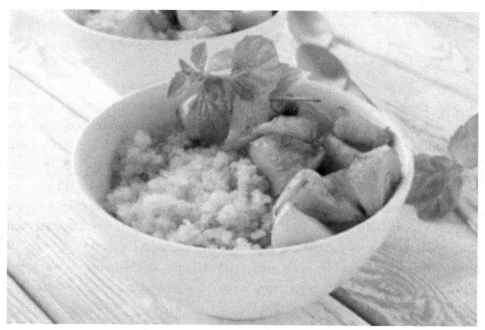

Preparation Time: 5 mins
Serves: 2

Ingredients:

Quinoa Porridge:

- Raisins 2 Tbsp
- Quinoa dry 1/2 cup
- Almond milk, unsweetened 1 cup

49

- Vanilla extract 1 tsp
- Cinnamon 1/4 tsp
- Cardamom 1/8 tsp

Sautéed Apples:

- Cinnamon 1/4 tsp
- Apple, chopped 1 large
- Coconut oil 1 tbsp

Method:
Rinse dried quinoa well to remove dirt and the outer layer of "saponins." Don't neglect this step; it will help you get rid of any bitterness. In a saucepan, combine rinsed quinoa, milk, vanilla, cardamom, cinnamon, raisins. Stir everything together well. Bring to a boil in a large saucepan over high heat. Cover and lower heat after the water has reached a boil. Allow for a 15-minute simmer or till all liquid has been absorbed. Turn off the heat and let the pot steam (covered) for a few minutes. Heat the coconut oil in another separate skillet over medium heat while the quinoa is cooking. Sprinkle with cinnamon and apple bits. Toss everything together and simmer for approximately 10 mins, or till the vegetables are gently browned and soft. To ensure consistent browning, stir every minute or two. Serve it in cooked quinoa in bowls with apples that have been sautéed. Enjoy!

Nutrition:
Calories: 229.3 kcal
Fats: 3.2 g
Proteins: 6.1 g
Carbs: 35.6 g

22. Vegetarian Sushi Cups

Preparation Time: 40 mins
Serves: 8

Ingredients:

Rice cups:

- Nonstick spray
- Sushi rice 1 cup
- Rice vinegar 3 tablespoons

Filling:

- Sesame seeds 2 tablespoons
- Sesame oil 1 teaspoon
- Soy sauce 2 tablespoons
- Rice vinegar 1 tablespoon
- Sriracha ½ teaspoon
- Garlic 1 clove, minced
- Grated fresh ginger 2 teaspoons
- European cucumber 1⅓ cups diced
- Peeled and diced 1 cup carrot
- Avocado 1 halved
- Green onions, 3 thinly sliced
- Chopped fresh cilantro 2 tablespoons

Method:

Bring the rice and 113 cups of water to a boil in a medium saucepan. Reduce heat to low, cover the saucepan, and simmer for 17 to 20 minutes, or till the rice has absorbed all of the water. Place the rice in a medium mixing basin and add the rice vinegar, constantly stirring till the rice is sticky enough yet to stay together when pressed. Spray a 12-cup muffin tin with nonstick spray before lining each cavity with parchment paper. Evenly distribute the rice among the muffin pan's chambers, pushing it into the bottom and up the edges to form compact rice cups. Refrigerate for 30 mins before serving. Meanwhile, whisk the sesame oil, rice vinegar, soy sauce, sriracha, garlic, and ginger in a medium mixing bowl. Cucumber, avocado, green onions, carrot, cilantro, and sesame seeds should all be combined. Lift the rice cups out of the pan using paper. Remove the paper from the rice cups and place them on a big dish. Fill the rice cups halfway with the veggie mixture. Enjoy!

Nutrition:
Calories: 89 kcal
Fats: 0 g
Proteins: 2 g
Carbs: 19 g

23. Butternut Mac And 'Cheese' With Smoky Shiitake 'Bacon.'

Preparation Time: 30 mins
Serves: 6

Ingredients:

Smoky shiitake 'bacon':

- Garlic powder ¼ teaspoon
- Shiitake mushrooms, 1 cup (4 ounces) stemmed and thinly sliced
- Olive oil 2 tablespoons
- Smoked paprika ¼ teaspoon

Mac and 'cheese':

- Smoked paprika, for serving
- Peeled and cubed 5 cups (20 ounces) butternut squash
- Olive oil 2 tablespoons
- Black pepper freshly ground
- Elbow macaroni 1 pound
- Raw cashews ½ cup
- Garlic 1 clove
- Dried rosemary ½ teaspoon

Method:
Preheat oven to 375 degrees Fahrenheit. Toss the mushrooms along with the

olive oil on a wide-rimmed baking sheet. Arrange the mushrooms in a single layer on the baking sheet. Cook, turning periodically with a spatula, till gently browned and extremely crisp, 20 to 30 mins on the center rack of the oven. Remove mushrooms from the oven and combine them with the smoked paprika and garlic powder, seasoning with salt and pepper to taste. Keep at room temperature for up to 3 days in an airtight container. Preheat oven to 400 ° degrees Fahrenheit. Toss the squash and the olive oil on a small cookie sheet and season with the pepper & 14 tsp of salt. Roast for 30 minutes, stirring regularly with a spatula until fork-tender. Over high heat, bring a big pot of generously salted water to a boil. Cook the macaroni until it is al dente, as directed on the packet. Drain the spaghetti and put it back in the saucepan, but turn off the heat. Blend the butternut squash, water, cashews, garlic, rosemary, and the remaining 2 tablespoons salt in a blender. Blend on high for 2 minutes, or until completely smooth. Toss the sauce with the noodles in the saucepan to coat. Season with salt and pepper to taste. If the sauce is too dense, add 1 tablespoon of water at a time until it reaches the appropriate consistency. Dust each plate with smoked paprika and smoky shiitake "bacon". Enjoy!

Nutrition:
Calories: 71 kcal
Fats: 7 g
Proteins: 1 g
Carbs: 2 g

24. Rainbow Collard Wraps with Peanut Butter Dipping Sauce

Preparation Time: 30 mins
Serves: 4

Ingredients:

Wraps:

- Mint leaves ½ cup
- Collard green leaves 4 large
- Hummus ½ cup
- Carrots, 4 peeled and cut into matchsticks
- English cucumber, 1 cut into matchsticks
- Avocados, 2 thickly sliced
- Red cabbage, shredded ½
- Basil leaves ½ cup

Dipping sauce:

- Garlic powder 1 teaspoon
- Peanut butter ½ cup
- Sweet chili sauce 2 tablespoons
- Soy sauce or tamari 2 tablespoons
- Rice vinegar ¼ cup

Method:
Bring a large saucepan of salted water to a boil, then blanch the collard leaves for 30 seconds in it. Using paper towels, pat dry. Trim away the thick, rough section of the stalk from one collard leaf at a time. Place 2 tablespoons of hummus in the middle of one of the leaves. Add a quarter of the carrots, avocado slices, cucumbers, and cabbage, as well as 2 teaspoons basil and mint each. Fold the leaf inwards toward the filling (as if folding a tortilla or wrap), then roll the contents securely within the leaf. Continue with the rest of the leaves and filling. Each wrap should be cut in half. Combine the peanut butter, soy sauce, sweet chili sauce, rice vinegar, and garlic powder in a medium mixing bowl. Serve the wraps right away with the dipping sauce, or keep them in the refrigerator firmly wrapped for up to 2 days. Enjoy!

Nutrition:
Calories: 264 kcal
Fats: 18 g
Proteins: 7 g
Carbs: 25 g

25. Curried Quinoa Chickpea Burgers

Preparation Time: 30 mins
Serves: 4

Ingredients:

- Curry powder 1 tsp
- Cooked and cooled quinoa 1 cup
- Chickpeas 1 15-oz can
- Avocado or coconut oil 1 tbsp

Potatoes:

- Harissa paste 2 tbsp
- Diced, peeled yellow potatoes 1 1/2 cups small
- Avocado or coconut oil 1 tbsp
- Curry powder 1 tsp
- Water 3-4 tbsp
- Raw or roasted cashews 2/3 cup
- Fresh minced ginger 2 tbsp (skin removed)
- Garlic, minced 4 cloves

Method:

Prepare your quinoa immediately if you haven't already. Preheat the oven to 375 degrees Fahrenheit (190 C). Toss rinsed dried chickpeas with oil, salt, & curry powder on a parchment-lined baking sheet. Cook for 20 minutes, or until the chickpeas are cracked and dry to the touch. Remove the chickpeas from the oven & place them on a plate to cool. Keep the oven turned on.

Meanwhile, combine diced potatoes (smaller / bite-size) with oil, salt, & curry powder in a rimmed, oven-safe medium pan. Cook for 4 mins with the lid on. Reduce the heat to medium-low, add the water, and cover once more. Cook until the potatoes are soft and browned on the edges. Then remove from heat and mash with a fork or potato masher until almost creamy. Remove from the equation. To make a semi-loose dough, combine cooked chickpeas, cashews, serrano pepper (optional), ginger, harissa paste, garlic, curry powder, and cilantro (optional) in a food processor. Then add the cooked/cooled quinoa & pulse to incorporate until you get a textured dough (not a purée). Add mashed potatoes to the mixture in a mixing basin. Stir to blend (do not overmix the potatoes in the food processor; they will get sticky if overmixed). Taste and adjust the seasonings as required, adding more curry powder for a stronger curry taste, salt for a saltier flavor, or harissa paste for a spicy kick. Form the mixture into discs approximately 3/4-inch in height by dividing it into 2/3-cup sections. Over medium heat, preheat the medium rimmed skillet (from earlier). Add a little oil and the burgers to the pan once it's heated, and cook for 2-3 minutes, or until the bottom side is golden brown. Transfer the pan to the oven and bake for 12-15 mins. Serve on a regular bun, with naan, atop a salad, or folded in a butter lettuce leaf as a side dish. Enjoy!

Nutrition:
Calories: 392 kcal
Fats: 18.5 g
Proteins: 12 g
Carbs: 46.8 g

26. Baked Apples

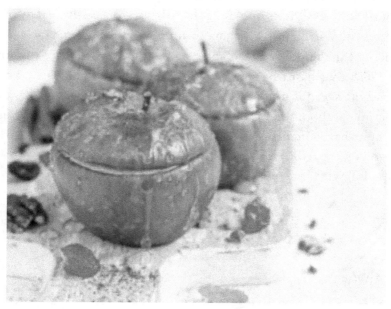

Preparation Time: 20 mins
Serves: 4

Ingredients:

- Melted coconut oil for drizzling
- Whole rolled oats ½ cup + 2 tablespoons
- Almond flour ½ cup
- Brown sugar ⅓ cup
- Crushed walnuts ¼ cup
- Apple pie spice ½ teaspoon
- Firm coconut oil ¼ cup
- Apples, 4 cored and halved

- Vanilla ice cream, for serving

Method:
Preheat oven to 375 degrees Fahrenheit.To make the topping, follow these steps: Combine the oats, walnuts, apple pie spice, almond flour, brown sugar, and salt in a small mixing basin. Work the hard coconut oil into the mixture with your hands until it crumbles. If the mixture is excessively dry, trickle in a few drops of water until it begins to hold together when pinched. Scoop out a piece of the middle of each apple half with a spoon. Place the apples in a baking dish that hasn't been buttered. Drizzle melted coconut oil over the apples and massaged it in. Bake for 10 mins after covering with foil. Uncover and pour liberal spoonfuls of the topping onto each half. Bake for 20 mins, or till the apples have softened as well as the topping is crisp, drizzling a little extra coconut oil on top. Allow it cool for a few minutes before serving with vanilla ice cream. Enjoy!

Nutrition:
Calories: 156 kcal
Fats: 3.3 g
Proteins: 0.6 g
Carbs: 34 g

27. Blistered Shishito Peppers

Preparation Time: 5 mins
Serves: 4

Ingredients:

- Tamari, for serving
- Shishito peppers 8 ounces
- Toasted sesame oil for drizzling
- Sesame seeds, for sprinkling
- Peanut sauce, for serving

Method:

A big cast iron skillet should be heated to high heat. Cook, stirring regularly, until the peppers are tender and scorching, approximately 6 to 8 mins in a dry skillet. Keep the peppers in a single layer as you work to ensure continuous contact with the hot pan. Drizzle sesame oil over the peppers and season with sesame seeds. To dip, serve with tamari & peanut sauce. Enjoy!

Nutrition:
Calories: 180 kcal
Fats: 8 g
Proteins: 6 g
Carbs: 29 g

28. Red Sangria

Preparation Time: 15 mins
Serves: 8

Ingredients:

- Cointreau ¼ to ½ cup
- Granny smith 1
- Orange, 1 thinly sliced, then sliced into quarters
- 1 lime, thinly sliced
- Raspberries ⅓ cup
- Tempranillo 1 (750 ml) bottle
- Orange juice ½ cup

Method:
In a large pitcher, combine the apple, orange, lime, & raspberries. Stir together wine, orange juice, & Cointreau. Refrigerate for at least 24 hours. In ice-filled cups, serve. Enjoy!

Nutrition:
Calories: 177 kcal
Fats: 0.1 g
Proteins: 0.5 g
Carbs: 15 g

29. Almond Flour Crackers

Preparation Time: 15 mins
Serves: 8

Ingredients:

- Almond flour 1 cup
- Flaxseed meal 2 tablespoons
- Water 4 tablespoons

Method:

Preheat the oven to 350 degrees Fahrenheit. Using parchment paper, line a baking sheet. Mix the flaxseed meal & water in a small bowl. Allow sitting for 10 mins, stirring occasionally. When the mixture is done, it will be gooey. This is the mixture's binder.

Flour made from almonds: You may either purchase almond flour or produce something similar at home. 1 and 1/4 cup raw almonds, ground into a fine powder or meal consistency in a blender/food processor.

To make the dough, follow these steps: Combine the flax mixture, almond flour, & optional spices in a medium-sized mixing bowl. Form the dough into a ball & set it on a flat surface coated with parchment paper to roll it out. Cover with some other parchment paper, flatten with your fingers, then roll out to approximately 1/8 inch thick using a rolling pin. The thinner the crackers are, the nicer and crispier they will be. Remove the top layer of paper and discard it. Cut into squares: Cut squares or diagonals into whichever size you choose using a pizza cutter or knife. Poke the middle of each cracker with a toothpick or tiny fork to enable steam to escape while baking (so they don't puff up). Add a pinch of coarse sea salt on top.

Bake: Line a baking sheet along with the parchment paper scraps. Bake for 10–15 minutes, carefully transferring each cracker to the baking sheet. After the first 10 mins, keep an eye on them and remove the ones done around the edges. They will gently deepen and get golden; you don't want it to go too dark or burn the taste. Allow cooling once completed. Enjoy!

Nutrition:
Calories: 150 kcal
Fats: 8 g
Proteins: 3 g
Carbs: 18 g

30. Quick N' Healthy Veggie Pasta Salad

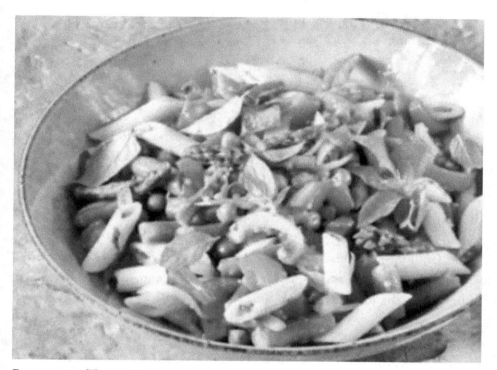

Preparation Time: 10 mins
Serves: 8

Ingredients:

- Zesty Garlic Lemon
- Bowtie pasta 16 oz.
- Cucumber, diced 1
- Red bell pepper, 1 cored and diced
- Orange bell pepper, 1 cored and diced

- Yellow bell pepper, 1 cored and diced
- Cherry tomatoes, 4 oz. Sliced in half
- Chickpeas (garbanzo beans), 1 can (15 oz.) Drained and rinsed

Dressing:

- Olive oil 1 – 2 tablespoons
- Garlic 4 large cloves, minced
- Lemons juice of 2 (about 1/4 – 1/3 cup)
- Dijon mustard 2 tablespoons

Method:
Cook the pasta as directed on the packet. Mix the garlic, dijon mustard, lemon juice, oil, and pepper in a small bowl to make the dressing. Remove from the equation.

Assemble the salad: Once the vegetables are ready, put the pasta, veggies, and dressing in a large mixing dish or the pot in which the pasta was cooked. Toss well to coat.

Chill: Chill for a few hours in the refrigerator or eat right away. Serve with a squeeze of lemon or a small sprinkle of Almond Parmesan cheese in separate dishes. Enjoy the small pleasures!

Nutrition:
Calories: 323 kcal
Fats: 3.5 g
Proteins: 11.2 g
Carbs: 62.7 g

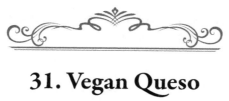

31. Vegan Queso

Preparation Time: 15 mins
Serves: 8

Ingredients:

- Chili powder 1/2 teaspoon
- raw cashews 1 cup
- Water 1/2 – 3/4 cup
- Garlic 1 clove
- Nutritional yeast 1 – 2 tablespoons
- Green chile peppers 1 4oz can
- Cumin 1/2 teaspoon

Method:
Soak the cashews in water. I prefer to soak my cashews in hot water for 5 mins before eating them. This allows them to soften and mix into pure creamy perfection. It's advised that you soak them in lukewarm water for up to 2 hrs to aid digestion. Soaking is not required. Combine the ingredients in a blender. Combine the cashews, water, garlic, chili powder, nutritional yeast, cumin, and salt in a blender cup. Blend for 1–2 minutes, pausing to scrape down the sides as required until creamy. As required, add extra water. Taste to see whether it's tasty. It should be warmed up (optional). Pour the vegan queso dip into an oven-safe dish, cover it with tin foil, and bake for 10–15 minutes at 350 degrees F. Warm in the microwave, uncovered, for 30 seconds at a time, stirring after each, until well warmed.
Serve: With your favorite tortilla chips or vegetable sticks, serve warm or at

room temperature. Top with sliced or diced jalapeno, red bell pepper, green onions, tomatoes, and cilantro. Enjoy!

Nutrition:
Calories: 145 kcal
Fats: 11 g
Proteins: 4 g
Carbs: 9.5 g

32. Greek Quinoa Salad

Preparation Time: 15 mins
Serves: 6

Ingredients:

- Lemon juice of 1 large
- Dried quinoa, rinsed 1 cup
- Water 1 3/4 cups
- Garlic powder 1 teaspoon
- Chickpeas (garbanzo beans), 1 can (14 oz) drained and rinsed
- Grape tomatoes, 1 cup sliced in half
- English cucumber, diced 1 cup
- Red onion, diced 1/2
- Kalamata olives (about 1 cup), 1 jar (7 oz) pitted and sliced
- Loosely packed 1/4 cup fresh parsley, chopped
- Fresh dill, 3 tablespoons chopped

Method:
Quinoa: Using a fine-mesh sieve, rinse the quinoa. Bring the water, quinoa, and garlic powder to a boil in a medium-sized saucepan. Cover and cook for 15 minutes on low heat. Remove the pan from the heat, cover, and set aside for 10–15 minutes. Using a fork, fluff the mixture. You can also prepare this Quinoa in the Instant Pot.Toss in the chickpeas, cucumber, onion, tomatoes, olives, and parsley after the quinoa is done. Mix thoroughly. Season with salt, freshly cracked pepper, and 1 big lemon juice. Serve over arugula or on its own. With pepperoncini and a squeeze of lemon juice on top, it's delicious. If

desired, drizzle with extra virgin olive oil. Season with salt and pepper to taste. This meal may be served hot, cold, or room temperature. Enjoy!

Nutrition:
Calories: 221.5 kcal
Fats: 8.1 g
Proteins: 7.1 g
Carbs: 30 g

33. Pozole (Posole Verde)

Preparation Time: 10 mins
Serves: 6

Ingredients:

- 1 – 2 juicy limes
- Olive oil 1 tablespoon
- Onion, diced 1 large
- Jalapeno, diced 1 large
- Garlic 3 – 4 cloves, minced
- Cumin 1 heaping teaspoon
- Oregano 1 heaping teaspoon
- Hominy drained and rinsed 1 can (25 – 28 oz)
- Pinto beans, 2 cans drained and rinsed
- Tomatillos (about 1 lb.), 6 medium husks removed
- Vegetable broth 4 cups low-sodium

Method:
Heat the oil/water in the Instant Pot, then add the onion & simmer for 5 minutes. Cook for 1-minute longer, or until aromatic, after adding the garlic, jalapeño, cumin, oregano, salt, and pepper. Combine pinto beans, tomatillos, hominy, and vegetable broth in a large mixing bowl. Cover with the lid and lock it in place. Set a valve to the SEALED position. Set the Pot to HIGH pressure and set the timer to 20 minutes manually. Allow 10 minutes for natural release before turning the valve to VENTING to remove any leftover steam. Season with lime juice and salt & pepper to taste. Enjoy!

Nutrition:
Calories: 313 kcal
Fats: 14 g
Proteins: 30 g
Carbs: 16 g

34. Farro (No-Fuss Recipe)

Preparation Time: 1 min
Serves: 4

Ingredients:

- Water 3 – 7 cups
- Farro 1 cup

Method:
Use 7 cups of water with a filter. Use 3 cups of water if you don't have a filter. Farro, water, and salt for pearled + semi-pearled farro Set the pressure cooker on HIGH for 7 mins for al dente farro (excellent for salads) or mins for softer farro. Set the valve to the SEALING position. After cooking, either do a rapid release or wait 5 mins before releasing pressure.

Whole farro: Combine farro, water, and salt in a high-pressure cooker. Cook on HIGH for 10 minutes, then turn the valve to SEALING. Allow for a 5-minute natural release before applying pressure. Adjust the water with or without the strainer & cook for 1 minute on LOW pressure with the valve set to SEAL. Allow for a 5-minute natural discharge. After you've finished cooking the farro, give it a thorough rinse under cold or warm running water. Salads, casseroles, nourish bowls, soups, and more may all benefit from this versatile ingredient. Enjoy!

Nutrition:
Calories: 200 kcal
Fats: 0 g

Proteins: 7 g
Carbs: 37 g

35. American Goulash

Preparation Time: 10 mins
Serves: 6

Ingredients:

- Elbow pasta 2 cups (about 8 oz.)
- Oil 2 tablespoons
- Tempeh, crumbled 2 (8oz.)
- Packages Onion, diced 1 large
- Pepper and fresh parsley
- Garlic, minced 4 cloves
- Green bell peppers, 2 cored, seedsdiced tomatoes 1 can (28oz.)
- Tomato sauce 1 can (14oz.)
- Dried oregano, 1 1/2 teaspoons
- EACH basil and paprika
- Bay leaves 2
- Red pepper flakes 1/4 teaspoon
- Vegetable broth 3 1/2 – 4 cups

Method:

Saute: In a large saucepan, boil the water/oil over medium heat, add the tempeh, onion, and bell pepper, and saute for 5–7 minutes, until onions are tender and tempeh is gently browned. Cook for another minute after adding the garlic.

Simmer: Combine the diced tomatoes, oregano, tomato sauce, basil, paprika, bay leaves, & red pepper flakes, as well as the water/veggie broth, and bring to a simmer. Bring to a boil, then cover, lower heat to low, and cook for 15 minutes. Cook for another 10 minutes, or until the pasta is cooked, often stirring to prevent the spaghetti from sticking to the bottom. Taste for seasoning, then seasons with extra salt and pepper as needed. Serve in separate dishes with a sprinkling of chopped fresh parsley on top. Enjoy!

Nutrition:
Calories: 333 kcal
Fats: 4.9 g
Proteins: 20.6 g
Carbs: 51.5 g

36. Roasted Butternut Squash Salad

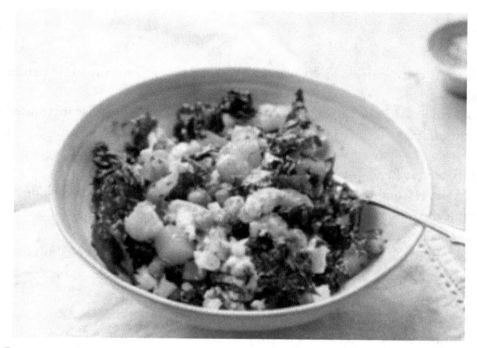

Preparation Time: 10 mins
Serves: 6

Ingredients:

- Salad mix of choice 8 oz.
- Butternut squash 1 medium
- Olive oil 1 tablespoon
- Pure maple syrup 1 tablespoon
- Dried cranberries 1/4 – 1/3 cup
- Pepitas (pumpkin seeds) 2 – 4 tablespoons

Shallot vinaigrette:

- Dijon 2 teaspoons
- Olive oil 2 tablespoons
- Water 2 tablespoons
- Shallot, minced 2 tablespoons
- Apple cider vinegar 1 tablespoon

Method:
Preheat the oven to 425 °F. Use parchment paper to line a roasting pan or gently oil it.
Squash Roast: Toss squash with olive oil & maple syrup before roasting. Spread butternut squash in a single layer on a baking sheet and season with pepper to taste. Cook, stirring halfway through, for 30 minutes, or till squash is fork-tender. Remove from the oven and set aside to cool.
Dressing: Combine the olive oil, vinegar, and mustard in a small bowl. Blend until the mustard is completely emulsified. Whisk in the water shallots, salt, and pepper until well mixed. Remove from the equation.
Assemble: Fill your serving dish along with your favorite salad, then top with butternut squash, cranberries, and pepitas. Serve with a drizzle of dressing on top. Enjoy!

Nutrition:
Calories: 82 kcal
Fats: 3.5 g
Proteins: 2 g
Carbs: 22 g

37. Cornbread

Preparation Time: 5 mins
Serves: 9

Ingredients:

- Lemon juice of 1 small
- Yellow cornmeal 1 cup
- Flour 1 cup
- Baking powder 1 tablespoon
- Organic sugar 1/3 cup
- Unsweetened almond milk 1 cup
- Olive oil 1/3 cup

Method:
Preheat the oven to 400 °F. Grease an 8- or 9" square baking pan lightly.
Wet & Sugar: Whisk the lemon juice, sugar, milk, and oil in a medium mixing bowl (or a 2-cup measuring cup). Set aside for 5–7 minutes, stirring periodically.
Dry: Combine the cornmeal, baking powder, flour, and salt in a large mixing dish.
Mix: When the oven is hot, put the wet and dry ingredients in a mixing bowl and whisk until smooth. Overmixing should be avoided. Pour batter into the prepared baking dish and bake. Preheat the oven to 350°F and bake the baking dish for 25 minutes, or lightly browned on top and cooked through in the middle. To check for doneness, stick a toothpick in the middle, and it should come out clean. Allow it to cool somewhat before slicing & serving. With chili,

soups, or stews, serve cornbread and vegan butter and homemade chia jam on the side. Enjoy!

Nutrition:
Calories: 94 kcal
Fats: 2.7 g
Proteins: 1.9 g
Carbs: 15 g

38. Macaroni Salad

Preparation Time: 10 mins
Serves: 12

Ingredients:

- Fresh dill, chopped 1/4 cup
- Elbow pasta 1 lb.
- Red onion, diced 1/2
- Red bell pepper, 1 cored and diced
- Carrot (about 1 cup), 1 large peeled and diced
- Celery (about 1 cup), 2 stalks diced
- Frozen peas, thawed 1 1/2 cups

Macaroni Dressing:

- Pepper 1/2 teaspoon
- Vegan mayo 1 cup
- Apple cider vinegar 1/4 cup
- Dijon 1 heaping tablespoon
- Pure maple syrup 1 tablespoon

Method:
Pasta: Cook elbow macaroni noodles till they are al dente, as directed on the packet. To stop the noodles from cooking, drain them and rinse them in cold water.
Dressing: Mix the ingredients for the creamy sauce in a small dish.
Assemble: Combine the pasta, onion, celery, bell pepper, carrots, peas, and dill

in a large mixing dish or the pot in which the pasta was cooked. Overtop, pour the creamy sauce and toss thoroughly to coat. Refrigerate the salad till ready to serve. Enjoy!

Nutrition:
Calories: 207 kcal
Fats: 9.5 g
Proteins: 3.7 g
Carbs: 26 g

39. Cream Cheese

Preparation Time: 15 mins
Serves: 1

Ingredients:

- Apple cider vinegar 1 teaspoon
- Raw cashews 1 + 1/2 cup
- Water 1/2 cup
- Lemon juice 3 tablespoons (about 2 – 3 small lemons)

Optional add-ins:

- Jalapeno, 1 small seeds removed and minced
- Fresh chives, chopped 3 tablespoons

Method:
Soak cashews: Place cashews in a bowl of boiling water & soak for 5–10 minutes. Alternatively, immerse them in cold water for 2–3 hours. Digestion will be aided by soaking.
Mix: Using a high-powered blender or a small personal blender, combine all of the ingredients in the cup of your choice and blend until smooth, scraping down the sides as needed. Stir in the optional add-ins if using. You may eat the vegan cream cheese straight away or refrigerate it before serving. Enjoy!

Nutrition:
Calories: 99 kcal
Fats: 10 g

Proteins: 2 g
Carbs: 2 g

40. Radish and Cucumber Salad

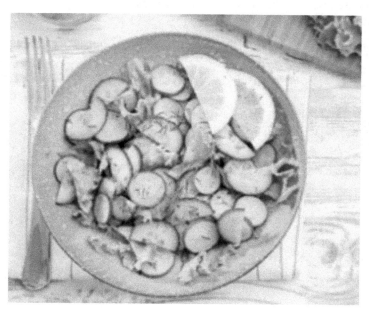

Preparation Time: 10 mins
Serves: 3

Ingredients:

- Apple cider vinegar 4 tablespoons
- Cucumber (about 2 cups), 1 thinly sliced
- Radishes (about 2 cups), 1 bunch thinly sliced
- Red onion (about 1/4 cup), 1/8 finely diced
- Fresh dill 3 tablespoons
- Chickpeas, 1 can (14oz) drained and rinsed
- Olive oil 1 – 2 tablespoons

Method:
Wash the cucumbers and radishes before using them. Remove the end and finely slice. To make eating simpler, cut the bigger chunks in half. Drain & rinse the chickpeas, then dice the red onion. Toss the cucumber, radish, chickpeas, dill, oil, apple cider vinegar, and pepper together in a large mixing basin. To taste, add additional dill, salt, and pepper. Enjoy!

Nutrition:
Calories: 194 kcal
Fats: 7.2 g
Proteins: 7.3 g
Carbs: 27 g

41. Apple, Beet, Carrot & Kale Salad

Preparation Time: 15 mins
Serves: 3

Ingredients:

- Cranberries 1/3 cup - 56g
- Apple 1 large
- Beets, 2 peeled and julienned
- Carrots, julienned 1 1/2 cups - 173g
- Curly kale leaves, 3 – 4 center vein

Orange Dressing:

- Onion powder 2 dashes
- Orange juice 4 tablespoons
- Apple cider vinegar 1 tablespoon
- Dijon mustard 2 teaspoons

Method:
To make the dressing, whisk together the orange juice, dijon mustard, apple cider vinegar, onion powder, salt, and pepper in a small bowl. Set them aside. Salad: In a large mixing basin, combine the prepped apple, beet, carrots, kale, and cranberries. Pour the dressing over the top & toss to coat. Serve in separate bowls with a sprinkling of pepitas and sunflower seeds as a garnish. Enjoy!

Nutrition:
Calories: 196 kcal

Fats: 3.9 g
Proteins: 6.5 g
Carbs: 34.8 g

42. Portobello Fajitas

Preparation Time: 10 mins
Serves: 3

Ingredients:

- Smoked paprika 1 teaspoon
- Olive oil 1 tablespoon
- Portobello mushrooms 2
- Onion, sliced 1/2 large
- Bell peppers sliced 3
- Garlic powder 3/4 teaspoon
- Cumin 1 teaspoon

Method:
Heat the oil or water in a large pan over medium heat, then throw in the peppers, cumin, smoky paprika, onions, garlic powder, and salt. Add the mushrooms and cook, occasionally turning, until the peppers & portobellos are tender, approximately 10 – 15 minutes. The avocado may be mashed or sliced. I mashed mine & added 1 lime juice, 2 tablespoons sliced jalapeño, and a big teaspoon of salt. Layer the mushroom-pepper mixture on each tortilla, then top it with avocado & cilantro. Squeeze a lime over the top. Enjoy!

Nutrition:
Calories: 304.6 kcal
Fats: 14.9 g
Proteins: 8 g

Carbs: 39.8 g

43. Baked Sweet Potato Wedges

Preparation Time: 10 mins
Serves: 2-3

Ingredients:

- Chipotle powder, 1 teaspoon optional
- Sweet potatoes 5 – 6 small
- Olive oil 1 – 2 tablespoons

Method:
Preheat the oven to 425 °F. Use parchment paper, line a rimmed baking sheet. Alternatively, gently butter a baking sheet. The sweet potatoes should be washed and dried. Any blemishes should be removed. Cut potatoes lengthwise into quarters and then cut them into smaller pieces as desired, ideally no more than 1 inch thick. Place on a baking sheet, sprinkle with olive oil and mix well. Arrange potatoes in a thin layer and season with salt and your favorite spice or herb. Place the baking sheet on the center rack of the oven and bake for 25–30 minutes, rotating once or twice. Remove from oven, allow to cool for a few minutes before serving with chopped parsley as well as garlic aioli. The ideal way to eat them is just out of the oven, but they're also good cold. If there are any leftovers, they will be OK the following day. Keep leftovers refrigerated for up to 5 days in an airtight container. Enjoy!

Nutrition:
Calories: 152.5 kcal
Fats: 0.5 g

Proteins: 2.9 g
Carbs: 35 g

44. Sonoma Chickpea 'Chicken' Salad

Preparation Time: 15 mins
Serves: 6

Ingredients:

- Pecans, roughly chopped 1/2 – 2/3 cup
- Chickpeas 2 cans (14 oz.)
- Seedless grapes, 1 1/2 cups sliced in half
- Celery ribs, diced 1/2 heaping cup

Creamy Poppy Seed Dressing:

- Garlic & onion powder
- Tahini 4 tablespoons
- Apple cider vinegar 2 tablespoons
- Pure maple syrup 1 tablespoon
- Dijon 2 teaspoons
- Poppy seeds 2 teaspoons

Method:

To make the dressing, put all of the ingredients in a small mixing dish. To thin, add water as required. Remove from the equation. Chickpea, Grape, Pecan, and Celery Salad: In a medium mixing/serving dish, combine chickpeas, pecans, grapes, and celery. Toss with the dressing to coat. Chickpea Salad (ideal for sandwiches): Place chickpeas in a medium mixing basin and mash 2/3 – 3/4 of them with the back of a fork and spoon. Toss in the grapes, pecans, or celery, then drizzle with the dressing and toss well. Chill or serve at room temperature.

Serve with leafy greens to make wraps, sandwiches, or just as a side dish. Enjoy!

Nutrition:
Calories: 295 kcal
Fats: 14.7 g
Proteins: 10.5 g
Carbs: 33.9 g

45. Balela Salad

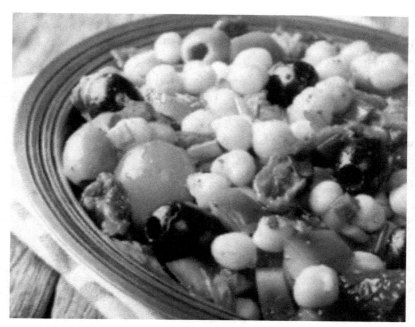

Preparation Time: 10 mins
Serves: 6

Ingredients:

- Lemon juice of 1 large
- Chickpeas (garbanzo beans), 2 cans (14 oz.) Drained and rinsed
- Black beans, 1 can (14 oz.) Drained and rinsed
- Roma tomatoes, 2 firm seeds removed and diced
- Red onion, diced 1/2
- English cucumber, diced 1/2
- Garlic, minced 3 cloves

- Fresh mint, chopped 2 tablespoons
- Fresh parsley, chopped 1/4 cup
- Sumac 1 teaspoon
- Olive oil 3 – 4 tablespoons

Method:

In a large mixing basin, combine the chickpeas, onion, cucumber, black beans, tomatoes, garlic, mint, and parsley. Add the sumac, olive oil, juice of lemon and pepper to taste. To blend, whisk everything together well. Serve refrigerated or at room temperature. Keep leftovers refrigerated for up to 5 days in an airtight container. This salad is delicious served on pita bread with hummus and arugula topped on top. You could also toss in a huge bunch of arugula & serve it with pita bread & hummus on the side. Enjoy!

Nutrition:

Calories: 281 kcal

Fats: 10.3 g

Proteins: 12.6 g

Carbs: 38.1 g

46. Banana Boats

Preparation Time: 5 mins
Serves: 1

Ingredients:

- Cacao nibs
- 1 per person bananas
- Natural peanut butter
- Goji berries
- Hemp hearts
- Shredded coconut

Method:
Bananas should be peeled and cut in half lengthwise. Layer your bananas, cut side up, beginning with the nut butter and working your way up. Then, in whichever sequence you desire, add the other ingredients. Enjoy!

Nutrition:
Calories: 136 kcal
Fats: 2 g
Proteins: 1 g
Carbs: 32 g

47. Spanish Vegan Paella

Preparation Time: 20 mins
Serves: 6

Ingredients:

- Lemon wedges, to serve
- Saffron or turmeric 1/2 heaping teaspoon
- Olive oil 2 tablespoons
- Yellow onion, 1 large thinly sliced
- Bell peppers 2 (red, orange or yellow)
- Garlic, minced 4 cloves
- Green beans 1 1/2 cups
- Tomatoes, 1 lb. (16 oz)
- Smoked paprika 1 1/2 teaspoons
- Red pepper flakes, 1 teaspoon optional
- Bay leaves 2 – 3
- Short grain rice 1 1/2 cups
- Vegetable broth 3 1/2 cups low-sodium
- Artichoke hearts in water, 1 can/jar (14 oz) drained and quartered
- Green peas 1 cup (fresh or frozen, thawed)
- Parsley leaves, chopped to garnish

Method:

Saffron steeping: Place the saffron threads in a small basin with warm water and steep for 10 minutes. In a big wide, flat-bottomed pan or paella pan, heat olive oil/broth over medium heat. Cook, occasionally stirring, until the onions

& bell peppers are soft, approximately 5 minutes. Cook for another 3 minutes, often stirring, with the garlic, green beans, red pepper flakes, tomatoes, smoked paprika, and bay leaves. Cook for another 7 minutes or so for softer vegetables for 10 mins after adding the last ingredients. Add the rice, broth, saffron mixture/turmeric, and salt to the pot. Move the veggies around gently so that the rice falls to the pan's bottom as much as possible. Bring to a boil, then lower to medium-low heat and cook for 15 minutes, uncovered, at a constant moderate boil. The rice should not be stirred. If you're using a big paella pan (15 inches or more), flip it over the fire now and then to help the rice cook evenly. Stay in the kitchen & clean up so you can quickly adjust the pan if necessary. Add a bit more warm water/broth if liquids appear to be boiling off too soon. After 15 minutes of simmering, spread the peas & artichoke hearts on top and cook for an additional 5 minutes.

To steam, cover: Turn off the heat and cover with a kitchen towel or even another suitable cover for 10 minutes. This will enable the rice to absorb the residual liquid while also steaming the peas and warming the artichoke hearts and any additional optional ingredients listed below. When the rice is done, fluff it gently and serve. Before eating, toss off the bay leaves. To taste, season with salt, pepper, or extra paprika.

Serve: Serve with chopped parsley as a garnish. With a side of lush greens and a squeeze of lemon on top, this dish is ideal. Serve immediately from the pan or in separate bowls.

Nutrition:
Calories: 332.3 kcal
Fats: 8.7 g
Proteins: 9.3 g
Carbs: 50.4 g

48. Kale + Red Cabbage Slaw

Preparation Time: 10 mins
Serves: 2

Ingredients:

- Pepitas (pumpkin seeds) 2 tablespoons
- Tuscan kale 1 small bunch
- Red cabbage, shredded 1/2 head small
- Carrots, grated or julienned 1 – 2
- Red onion, thinly sliced 1/3
- Parsley leaves, 1/2 cup roughly chopped
- Hemp hearts 2 tablespoons
- Sunflower seeds 2 tablespoons

Dressing:

- Water 2 tablespoons
- Olive oil 1 tablespoon
- Dijon mustard 1 tablespoon
- Apple cider vinegar 1 tablespoon

Method:
Mix your dressing in a small dish and put it aside. Prepare the veggies and set them in a big mixing basin with the dressing. Toss to coat. Toss in the seeds one more. Allow the salad to sit for a few mins before serving to soften the greens. Enjoy!

Nutrition:
Calories: 113.3 kcal
Fats: 9.2 g
Proteins: 0.8 g
Carbs: 8.2 g

49. Hummus Veggie Wrap

Preparation Time: 5 mins
Serves: 3
Ingredients:

- Red pepper flakes, to taste
- Lavash bread 3
- Kale 1 bunch
- Red bell pepper, 1 sliced
- Yellow bell pepper, 1 sliced
- Carrots, 1 – 2 sliced
- Cucumber, 1 thinly sliced
- Hummus 3/4 cup

Method:
Spread hummus over a lavash bread (or tortilla) on a level surface, leaving an inch on both ends. Vegetables are layered on top. Wrap one end around the other and roll it up. Slice in half and eat right away or save for later. Enjoy!

Nutrition:
Calories: 740 kcal
Fats: 38 g
Proteins: 18 g
Carbs: 83 g

50. Raw Ginger Snaps

Preparation Time: 25 mins
Serves: 12

Ingredients:

- Nutmeg or ground cloves 1/8 teaspoon
- Oats, regular or quick 1 cup
- Raw almonds 1/2 cup
- Pure maple syrup 1/4 cup
- Ginger powder 1 1/2 teaspoons
- Unsulphured organic molasses 1 tablespoon
- Vanilla 1/2 teaspoon
- Cinnamon 1/4 teaspoon

Method:
Blend oats and almonds in the bowl of a food processor until a reasonably fine consistency is achieved; it doesn't have to be perfect. Add the other ingredients and mix for 1 minute, scraping down the sides as required, until well blended and a dough-like consistency is achieved. If you feel the mixture is too dry after adding additional oats or nuts/seeds, add water at a time until you get the correct consistency. Refrigerate the ingredients for approximately 20 minutes to help firm the dough for rolling.
Roll: Scoop up rounded teaspoons of dough with a measuring spoon and roll into 1 inch balls. Roll them in shredded coconut, cacao powder, cinnamon, or white sesame seeds to make the truffles seem complete. Enjoy!

Nutrition:
Calories: 87 kcal
Fats: 0 g
Proteins: 0 g
Carbs: 0 g

Conclusion

Plant-based diets have been linked to a variety of health advantages, including a lower risk of heart disease, cancer, obesity, diabetes, or cognitive decline. Transitioning to a more plant-based diet is also good for the environment. Whatever sort of whole-foods, plant-based diet you select, you will see a significant improvement in your health. Veganism is both a philosophy and a way of life. It has nothing to do with a person's diet.

People that consume plant-based diets do so for a variety of reasons, including health and the environment. Animal products may be excluded in varied degrees. Flexitarian, pescatarian, and vegan diets are all plant-based diets. There is evidence that eating a plant-based diet is good for both people and the environment.

To avoid deficiency, someone who wants to eat a plant-based diet must satisfy their nutritional needs. Many individuals are choosing to minimize or eliminate their use of animal products. While some individuals choose not to name their dietary choices, others identify as vegan or plant-based.

"Plant-based" usually refers to a diet that consists mostly of plant foods and contains little or no animal-derived items. Oils & processed packaged foods are also banned from a whole foods, plant-based diet.

Don't miss out!

Visit the website below and you can sign up to receive emails whenever Penny Tripp publishes a new book. There's no charge and no obligation.

https://books2read.com/r/B-A-HHOU-VLGAC

BOOKS 2 READ

Connecting independent readers to independent writers.

9 798201 464080